Samir Samaâli
Abir Hakiri
Rym Ghachem

Telemedicine in psychiatry

Samir Samaâli
Abir Hakiri
Rym Ghachem

Telemedicine in psychiatry

issues and prospects for an emerging medical practice in Tunisia

ScienciaScripts

Imprint

Cover image: www.ingimage.com

This book is a translation from the original published under ISBN 978-620-6-72355-4.

Publisher:
Sciencia Scripts
is a trademark of
Dodo Books Indian Ocean Ltd. and OmniScriptum S.R.L publishing group

120 High Road, East Finchley, London, N2 9ED, United Kingdom
Str. Armeneasca 28/1, office 1, Chisinau MD-2012, Republic of Moldova, Europe
Printed at: see last page
ISBN: 978-620-8-27039-1

TABLE OF CONTENTS

INTRODUCTION 2

METHODS 3

RESULTS 6

DISCUSSION 13

CONCLUSIONS 28

REFERENCES 30

APPENDICES 33

INTRODUCTION

The development of information and communication technologies (ICTs) has revolutionised the field of healthcare, leading to a transformation in the way care is delivered. Telemedicine is, by definition, the use of ICTs for medical purposes and consists of providing care at a distance. The scope of telemedicine covers a wide range of procedures. In 1997, the World Health Organisation (WHO) defined telemedicine as "that part of medicine which uses the transmission of medical information (images, reports, audio and video recordings) by telecommunication for the purpose of obtaining a diagnosis, specialist opinion, patient monitoring or therapeutic decision from a distance" (1).Around the world, the development of telemedicine has become a hot topic in the news in recent years, and its importance was particularly highlighted during the COVID-19 pandemic. Some healthcare systems had to rely on this form of medical practice to reduce transmission of the virus and maintain continuity of care (2).The practice of telemedicine in Tunisia was regulated by Law 2018-43 of 11 July 2018, which amended Law 91-21 of 13 March 1991 relating to the practice and organisation of the medical and dental professions (3,4). However, in order to specify the terms of application of this practice, Presidential Decree No. 318/2022 was recently published in the Journal Officiel de la République Tunisienne (JORT) on 8 April 2022 (5).In the Tunisian context, and despite the limited experience reported with telemedicine, there are no data on Tunisian doctors' adherence to this new emerging medical practice (6,7).Since psychiatry is a speciality in which the clinical interview plays a vital role both for diagnostic and therapeutic purposes, telemedicine may prove particularly applicable due to the absence of examination equipment. specific. Nevertheless, the intrusion of the machine into the doctor-patient relationship could jeopardise therapeutic communication and consequently alter the quality of this relationship.

In light of these new issues, we propose in this dissertation to :

-Assessing the knowledge, perception and acceptance of telemedicine among Tunisian psychiatrists and child psychiatrists

To raise the ethical and medico-legal issues that may arise from the practice of telemedicine in psychiatry in our Tunisian context.

METHODS

1. Type of study :

This was a descriptive cross-sectional study. The study took place over a period of one and a half months, from 15 November 2022 to 31 December 2022. The survey was conducted online using an electronic questionnaire designed on the Google Forms platform.

2. Participants:

Inclusion criteria :

- Tunisian psychiatrists and child psychiatrists practising in Tunisia in both the public and private sectors.
- Participants who agreed to take part in the survey.

Non-inclusion criteria :

- The doctors from other specialties medical surgical or biological specialities.
- Medical interns and externs.

Exclusion criteria :

- Tunisian psychiatrists and child psychiatrists practising outside Tunisia.

3. Conduct of the study :

Initially, we contacted the executive office of the ATPEP "Association tunisienne des psychiatres d'exercice privé", which provided us with the electronic contact details (a mailing list) of psychiatrists and child psychiatrists in free practice. We also obtained a list of the e-mail addresses of residents in psychiatry and child psychiatry, as well as those of psychiatrists and psychiatrists working in psychiatry. child psychiatrists from the Collège National de Psychiatrie et Pédopsychiatrie. The questionnaire was sent to 391 participants.

4. Drawing up the questionnaire :

In the absence of a structured and validated psychometric scale for evaluating knowledge of and attitudes towards telemedicine, we used a questionnaire drawn up by our team which met the needs of the survey. The questions were drawn up with reference to the Tunisian laws governing the practice of medicine in Tunisia, the recommendations of learned societies concerning the practice of telemedicine and telepsychiatry, and taking into account certain specific features of the Tunisian psychiatric care system. Thus, during the development of the questionnaire, our team based itself on the following references:

1. Presidential Decree no. 2022-318 of 8 April 2022, laying down the general conditions for the practice of telemedicine and the areas of its application (5) **(Appendix 2)**.

2. Tunisian Code of Medical Ethics (8).

3. Tunisian Penal Code (9).

4. The AETMIS (Agence d'Évaluation des Technologies et des Modes d'Intervention en Santé) recommendations and technological standards for telepsychiatry (10).

5. The ATA (American Telemedicine Association) recommendations for telemedicine practice in mental health (11).

6. The 2022 International Code of Medical Ethics of the WMA (Medical Association of Mondiale) (12).

7. Guide de bon usage de la télémédecine de la HAS (Haute Autorité de Santé) (13).

The questionnaire was designed according to a semi-structured model with 53 questions, including two clinical vignettes that lend themselves to ethical and legal discussion. The majority of questions were closed-ended with binary responses, 7 questions were multiple-choice and only the question in the second vignette was open-ended. General acceptance of telepsychiatry was assessed by a binary question with two answers: "favourable" or "unfavourable".

In addition to socio-demographic and professional data, the questionnaire included :

- Questions about the technological equipment available in the workplace

- Questions assessing knowledge of the law, the scope of telemedicine and existing recommendations

- Questions on the perception and representation of telemedicine and the usefulness of its use in Tunisian psychiatry and psychiatric care.

- Questions on ethical and legal issues

5. Bibliographical research :

We carried out a bibliographic search using the Pubmed and Science Direct search engines and Google Scholar. Mesh keywords (Medical Subjet headings) from the National Library of Medicine were combined: The words used were: Telemedicine, psychiatry, Ethic, Perception, Attitude, Legal aspects.

6. Statistical analysis :

The data were entered and analysed using SPSS software version 26. Simple frequencies and percentages were calculated for the qualitative variables. Means, extreme values (minimum and maximum) and standard deviations were determined for quantitative variables. Where there was no normality, medians and interquartiles were calculated. Comparisons of percentages on independent series were made using Pearson's chi-square test. Where this test was invalid, the two-tailed Fisher exact test was used. In all statistical tests, the significance level was set at 0.05.

7. Ethical considerations :

All participants were informed of the purpose of the study, the anonymity of participation and the possibility of refusing to participate. The study was approved by the Razi Hospital Ethics Committee **(Appendix 3)**.

RESULTS

1. Sample size :

During data collection, 70 participants replied to the questionnaire, corresponding to 17.9% of the doctors who had been contacted by e-mail. Among the participants who responded to the questionnaire, there were two psychiatrists who were practising abroad at the time of the study, so they were excluded. A total of 68 participants were included in the survey.

2. Socio-demographic and professional characteristics of the doctors surveyed :

The median age of the participants was 32±10 years. A female predominance (78%; n=53) was found with a sex ratio (male / female) of 0.28. Of the participants, 82% (n=56) practised in psychiatry and 18% (n=12) practised in child psychiatry. Half of the participants were residents (junior doctors) (50%, n=34). The practice sector was public in 69% (n=47) and private in 31% (n=21) of cases.The various socio-demographic and occupational characteristics of the study population are detailed in Table I.

Table I: Socio-demographic and professional data of the doctors surveyed

Age		32±10 years [24-71]
Gender	man	22%(n=15)
	woman	78%(n=53)
Number of years' professional experience		5±7 years
Speciality	Psychiatry	82%(n=56)
	Child psychiatry	18%(n=12)
Professional status	Resident	50%(n=34)
	University hospital assistant	13%(n=9)
	Associate Professor	6%(n=4)
	Professor	3%(n=2)
	Specialist	28%(n=19)
Current area of practice	Public	69%(n=47)
	Private	31%(n=21)
Place of work	Urban area	99%(n=67)
	Rural areas	1%(n=1)
Average time taken to obtain a	2 weeks	73%(n=50)
first appointment	1 month	15%(n=10)
	3 months	12%(n=8)
How to make an appointment	Paper diary	75%(n=51)
	Electronic diary	16%(n=11)
	Online electronic diary	16%(n=11)
	On-site secretary	40%(n=27)
Patient travelling more than 100	Yes	91%(n=62)
km (return journey) to consult you	No	9%(n=6)
Logistical impediment to	Yes	99%(n=67)
consultation	No	1%(n=1)
Reason(s) for cancellation of the	Geographical remoteness (absence	60%(n=41)
consultation	means of transport)	
	Constraints on the patient's work schedule when travelling Somatic problems	44%(n=30) 28%(n=19) 32%(n=22)

3. Use and availability of technological resources among the doctors surveyed :

The majority of participants (96%; n=65) had already used technology (telephone, e-mail, Facebook, WhatsApp and social networks) in their daily work. At the participants' workplaces, around half of them (53%; n=36) had a computer and only 28% (n=19) had high-speed internet access (at least 384 kilobits per second (kbps)) (Table II).

Table II: Use and availability of technological equipment among the doctors surveyed

Variables	Answers	Percentages (headcount)
Use of technology in professional practice	Yes No	96%(n=65) 4%(n=3)
Main professional use	Requests for advice Communication with the patient Communication with the patient's family	93%(n=63) 54%(n=37) 59%(n=40)
Crisis intervention by telephone	Yes No	72%(n=49) 28%(n=19)
Effectiveness of telephone intervention according to the doctor	Effective Ineffective	98%(48) 2%(n=1)
Type of technological equipment available at work	Broadband Internet (at least 384 kbps) Computer Camera Microphone Headset Smartphone Tablet	28% (n=19) 53%(n=36) 18%(n=12) 18%(n=12) 10%(n=7) 79%(n=54) 7%(n=5)

Kbps: Kilobits per second

4. Assessment of doctors' knowledge of telemedicine :

More than half the respondents (62%; n=42) were not aware of the various telemedicine procedures. More than two thirds of participants (73%; n=51) replied that they knew the definition of teleconsultation and 57% (n=39) of doctors were not aware of the existence of Presidential Decree-Law No. 318 / 2022 relating to the practice of telemedicine in Tunisia (Table III).

Table III: Knowledge of telemedicine among doctors surveyed

Questions	Response	Percentages(Numbers)
Knowledge of the various telemedicine procedures	Yes No	38%(n=26) 62%(n=42)
Definition of teleconsultation	Yes No	73%(n=51) 27%(n=19)
Definition of tele-expertise	Yes No	22% (n=15) 78%(n5=3)
Definition of remote medical monitoring	Yes No	41%(n=28) 59%(n=40)
Definition of remote medical assistance	Yes No	32%(n=22) 68%(n=46)
Definition of medical regulation	Yes No	32%(n=22) 68%(n=46)
Definition of electronic medical prescription	Yes No	59%(n=40) 41%(n=28)
Knowledge of Presidential Decree-Law No. 318 /2022 relating to the practice of telemedicine in Tunisia	Yes No	43%(n=29) 57%(n=39)
Knowledge of the procedure for practising telemedicine in Tunisia	n Yes No	18%(n=12) 82%(n=56)
Knowledge of good practice recommendations for telepsychiatry	Yes No	21%(n=14) 79%(n=54)
Possibility of issuing medical prescriptions (table B psychotropic drugs) via telemedicine	Yes No	59%(n=40) 41%(n=28)
Possibility of practising telemedicine with a patient abroad	Yes No	94%(n=64) 6%(n=4)

5. Benefits of training :

The majority (74%; n=50) of respondents felt that academic training in telemedicine was necessary. The main interest in this training concerned the application of telemedicine, which was highlighted by 62% (n=42) of doctors.

6. Perception and usefulness of telepsychiatry :

According to 88% of the doctors, telepsychiatry could be useful in the Tunisian health care system, and 94% (n=64) of them thought that telepsychiatry could facilitate access to care. Interest in the practice of telepsychiatry in public hospitals was expressed by 79% (n=54) of doctors. Telepsychiatry can alleviate the shortage of psychiatrists in disadvantaged regions, according to 78% of respondents (n=53). For 88% of participants, telepsychiatry can be applied to psychotherapeutic techniques (Table IV).

Table IV: Perception and usefulness of telepsychiatry according to the doctors surveyed

Questions	Answers	Percentages (Numbers)
The usefulness of telepsychiatry in the Tunisian healthcare system	Yes No	90%(n=61) 10%(n=7)
Telepsychiatry facilitates access to care	Yes No	94%(n=64) 6%(n=4)
Telepsychiatry is as much about	Yes	88%(n=60)
psychiatrists than free-lance psychiatrists	No	12%(n=8)
university hospitals		
Telepsychiatry is an alternative solution	Yes	82%(n=56)
for the underdevelopment of psychiatry in the	No	18%(n=12)
link		
The usefulness of telepsychiatry in public hospitals	Yes No	79%(n=54) 21%(n=14)
Telepsychiatry could be a solution for the	Yes	78%(n=53)
shortage of psychiatrists in the regions	No	22%(n=15)
disadvantaged		
Usefulness in the prison environment (for detained patients)	Yes No	74%(n=50) 26%(n=18)*
Telepsychiatry can be envisaged as :	Child psychiatry	59%(n=40)
	Adult psychiatry	96%(n=65)
	Geriatric psychiatry	75%(n=51)
Usefulness of telepsychiatry practice :	First contact	56%(n=38)
	During emergencies	43%(n=29)
	During patient follow-up	97%(n=54)
	(surveillance)	
Useful in :	Addictology	74%(n=50)
	Psychotherapeutic technique	88%(n=60)
	Managing suicidal crises	62%(n=42)
	Cognitive remediation	63%(n=43)
	Others :	
	follow-up after an initial consultation	1%(n=1)
	Teleconsultation and medical referrals	1%(n=1)

7. Ethical and medico-legal issues in telepsychiatry :

About half (56%; n=38) of the doctors thought that telemedicine risked dehumanizing the practice of psychiatry, and about a quarter (28%; n=19) of them replied that telepsychiatry did not respect the ethical principles of medicine in the Tunisian context. The majority of doctors (81%; n=55) replied that telepsychiatry was more prone to legal problems than traditional psychiatry (Table V).

Table V: Responses from doctors surveyed on ethical and medico-legal issues relating to telepsychiatry

Questions	Answers	Percentage (headcount)
Telepsychiatry risks dehumanising psychiatry	Yes No	56%(n=38) 44,1%(n=30)
Telepsychiatry alters the quality of psychiatric interviews	Yes No	35%(n=44) 65%(n=24)
Telepsychiatry has a negative impact on the quality of the doctor-patient relationship	Yes No	43%(n=29) 57%(n=39)
Telepsychiatry respects universal ethical principles in the Tunisian context	Yes No	72%(n=49) 28%(n=19)
Ethical principle that telepsychiatry does not respect in the Tunisian context	Autonomy Beneficence Non-maleficence Equity	6%(n=4) 3%(n=2) 6%(n=4) 13%(n=9)
Telepsychiatry is more prone to medico-legal problems than traditional psychiatry	Yes No	81%(n=44) 19%(n=13)
There is a greater risk of disclosure of medical confidentiality with telepsychiatry than with traditional psychiatry.	Yes No	49%(n=33) 51%(n=35)

8. Answers to thumbnails :

Vignette 1: When we asked the question about whether a patient being treated for bipolar disorder should be informed of the diagnosis of HIV serology (+), 72% (n=49) of respondents did not agree with communicating this information via teleconsultation.

Vignette 2: The situation of a patient, in suicidal crisis with a high suicidal risk, not resolved through teleconsultation, the responses have been grouped in the table below.

Table VI: Responses to Vignette 2

Answers	Percentage (Number)
-Contacting the family (close friends, support person)	47% (n=31)
-Ask the patient to have a face-to-face consultation as soon as possible	15% (n=10)
-Ask the patient to consult a psychiatric emergency unit	13% (n=9)
-Contact the public prosecutor	5% (n=3)
-Request hospitalisation under duress (HO, HDT)	13% (n=9)
-Prescribe a sedative treatment	1% (n=1)
-Continuing to manage suicidal crises from a distance	4% (n=3)
-Notify an ambulatory team	1% (n=1)
-Refusal of consultation for the management of a suicidal crisis and asking the patient to consult emergency services	1% (n=1)

HO = compulsory hospitalisation; HDT = hospitalisation at the request of a third party

9. Telepsychiatry membership :

The majority of participants (84%; n=57) were in favour of telepsychiatry. No association was found between support for telepsychiatry and gender (p=0.69), physician status (p=0.512), number of years in practice (p=0.834) or practice sector (p=1) (Table VII).

Table VII: Association between acceptance of telemedicine and professional and socio-demographic variables

Variables	Favourable opinion n=57	Negative opinion n=11	P
Gender male female	21%(n=12) 97%(n=45)	27%(n=3) 73%(n=8)	p=0,69
Junior doctor status Senior	47%(n=27) 53%(n=30)	64%(n=7) 36%(n=4)	p=0,512
Number of years' professional experience	6±7 years [1-40]	4±11 years [2-43]	p=0,834
Speciality Psychiatry Child psychiatry	82%(n=47) 18%(n=10)	82%(n=9) 18%(n=2)	p=1
Practice area Public Private	68%(n=39) 32%(n=18)	73%(n=8) 72%(n=3)	p=1

DISCUSSION

1. Main results :

In the present survey, the total number of participants was 68, divided into 50% senior doctors and 50% junior doctors (residents). Women predominated (78%; n=53). The median number of years of professional experience was 5±7 years. Of the participants, 82% (n=56) practised in psychiatry and 18% (n=12) in child psychiatry. The practice sector was public in 69% (n=47) and private in 31% (n=21) of cases. About half of the participants (53%; n=36) had a computer at work, but only 28% (n=19) had broadband internet access (at least 384 kbps). The majority (62%; n=42) were not familiar with the various telemedicine procedures. More than half (57%, n=39) of doctors are unaware of the existence of Presidential Decree No 318 / 2022 relating to the practice of telemedicine in Tunisia. Around half (56%; n=38) of doctors thought that telemedicine risked dehumanising the practice of psychiatry.The majority of doctors (81%; n=55) replied that telepsychiatry was more prone to legal problems than traditional psychiatry. According to 49% (n=33), telepsychiatry increases the risk of disclosure of medical confidentiality. Telepsychiatry alters the quality of the psychiatric interview according to 65% (n=44) of respondents, and has a negative impact on the quality of the doctor-patient relationship according to 43% (n=39). About a quarter of the participants (28%; n=19) replied that telepsychiatry does not respect the ethical principles of medicine in our Tunisian context. The majority of doctors (84%) were in favour of telepsychiatry. No association was found between support for telepsychiatry and the status of the doctor (p=0.512), the number of years of professional experience (p=0.834) and his or her area of practice (p=1).

2. Relevance and limitations of the study :

To our knowledge, this is the first Tunisian study to assess the knowledge of Tunisian doctors, in this case psychiatrists, about telemedicine. The main interest of this work lies in the evaluation of perceptions and knowledge of telemedicine among mental health professionals a few months after the publication of the decree-law relating to its practice. This study provides primary data on the interest of psychiatrists and child psychiatrists in this new medical practice. As the first Tunisian study to look at the issue of telemedicine among Tunisian psychiatrists, it was relevant to identify their training needs and to pinpoint certain concerns on the subject. Addressing the ethical and legal aspects of telepsychiatry from the point of view of its future practitioners will provide a better understanding of the new challenges that Tunisian psychiatrists may face.Nevertheless, this work has methodological limitations:The participation rate was low (<20%) and the sample size was not representative of all Tunisian psychiatrists and child psychiatrists in both the private and public sectors. In addition, the assessment of knowledge was non-objective and not validated by a reliable psychometric tool. In the absence of such a tool, we developed a questionnaire adapted to the study.

3. Assessment of knowledge of telemedicine :

More than half of the participants (57%, n=39) had not heard of the presidential decree-law relating to the practice of telemedicine in Tunisia and were therefore still unaware of the legal framework governing it. This lack of knowledge reflects, among other things, the lack of dissemination of the law and the lack of information among Tunisian doctors about the legal framework for the practice of telemedicine. This result can be partly explained by certain characteristicsIn addition, the period between the publication of the decree-law and our survey was relatively short (eight months), which may also help to explain this result. In addition, the period between publication of the decree-law and our survey was relatively short (8 months), which may also help to explain this result. Despite this fairly recent publication of the first decree implementing the law, it is important to stress that the concept of digital health in general is not so new in Tunisia. The first experience of telemedicine dates back to October 1996, when an occasional link was established between La Rabta hospital and the Paul Brousse hospital in Paris. Following this initiative, telemedicine was included by the Minister in his strategic IT plan, and the National Telemedicine Committee (CNT) was set up on 15 May 1996 (14).The establishment of a legal framework for the practice of telemedicine in Tunisia was initiated by Law 2018-43 of 11 July 2018, which made amendments to Law 91-21 of 13 March 1991 on the practice and organisation of doctors and dentists, by including telemedicine as a sixth type of medical act authorised for health professionals (3,4). However, in order to define the conditions of application of this new medical practice, Presidential Decree no. 318/2022 was published in the JORT on 8 April 2022. This decree sets out the general conditions for telemedicine and its areas of application. Table VIII illustrates the 29 articles divided into 4 chapters contained in Presidential Decree no. 318/2022 (5).

Table VIII: Chapters and sections of Presidential Decree-Law No. 318/2022 laying down the general conditions for the practice of telemedicine and its scope of application

Chapter	Title	Section/Article
Chapter 1:	General provisions	Article 2 □ Article 4
Chapter 2:	Areas of application for telemedicine	Article 5□ Article 7
Chapter 3:	General conditions for telemedicine practice	Section 1: Authorisation Article 8 □ Article 13 Section 2: Technical conditions Article 14□ Article 18 Section 3: Guarantees for the practice of medicine Article 19□ Article 23 Section 4: Terms of payment Article 24□ Article 25
Chapter 4:	Final and transitional provisions	Article 26□ Article 29

3.1. Areas of application for telemedicine :

A lack of knowledge was found among the doctors surveyed regarding the various telemedicine modalities, with the exception of teleconsultation, which 73% of them said they knew about. This result may be explained by the fact that teleconsultation is the telemedicine procedure most frequently used and widespread in our speciality.Telepsychiatry is the specific application of telemedicine in the field of mental health. It is even considered to be its oldest application, with the first teleconsultation experiments initiated in the United States in 1958 (15).In psychiatry, the most commonly used telemedicine procedures are teleconsultation and tele-expertise. In addition to these two areas, telemedicine has several other areas of application, including remote medical monitoring, remote medical assistance and medical regulation. The first chapter of the decree-law defines the various acts involved, as well as concepts relating to digital health such as electronic medical prescription and the medical platform.

3.2. Telemedicine and administrative requirements

Ignorance of the procedure for practising telemedicine was reported by 83% of doctors. This result highlights the need to provide information about the administrative issues involved and the conditions required to enable telemedicine to be practised.In a second chapter, the law sets out the general conditions for practising telemedicine: one section is dedicated to authorising the setting up of a platform, highlighting the requirement for two authorisations from the INPDP (national body for the protection of personal data) and an authorisation from the Minister of Health.Article 11 specifies that the telemedicine platform may only be used if the doctor concerned has entered into an agreement with the owner of the platform. If the doctor or dentist works in the private sector, his or her professional association must approve the agreement and inform the Ministry of Health. If the doctor works in the public sector, the agreement must be approved by the Ministry of Health.

3.3. Telemedicine and psychotropic drugs (Table B) :

According to 59% of participants, it is possible to issue a Table B prescription via telemedicine. This result further highlights the participants' lack of awareness of the law, since the method of dispensing medicines by pharmacies excluding table B medicines and psychotropic drugs subject to ministerial control as announced in article 18 of the decree-law.

3.4. Telemedicine and cross-border practice :

Contrary to the response from four participants, it is legally permitted to practise telemedicine on patients residing abroad. According to article 13, authorisation to practise medicine across borders must be granted following prior notification to the Ministry of Health and the relevant professional bodies.

3.5. Telemedicine and recommendations :

The majority of participants had never read the recommendations on telemedicine. However, these recommendations are essential to know, as they are designed to guide and direct doctors in their good practice, based on ethical guidelines, expert opinions, scientific data and established standards for data protection and the confidentiality of medical information (10-13).

4. The role of telemedicine training

The majority of doctors replied that training in telemedicine is necessary. Today, training is considered to be a key factor in the expansion of telemedicine and the removal of barriers to its implementation. One example of this is the strategy adopted by the United States. In order to successfully integrate telemedicine into the continuum of care in the United States, courses have been included in the curricula for medical studies with a view to effectively exploiting telemedicine technologies in students' future careers (16).

5. Representation and usefulness of telepsychiatry :

In the present study, despite a lack of knowledge, the majority of doctors expressed a favourable opinion of their adherence to telepsychiatry, indicating a positive perception of the use of information and communication technologies in their clinical practices. This result is consistent with that of a recent study carried out by Albarrak et al in Saudi Arabia to assess the knowledge and perception of telemedicine among doctors in different specialties. Most doctors had average knowledge of telemedicine technology, but they had a positive perception of it and were willing to adopt it in their clinical practice. The main obstacles to the practice of telemedicine mentioned in the study were the lack of appropriate training and the lack of coordination between information technology experts and clinicians (17).

In the present survey, the value of telemedicine in psychiatry was demonstrated independently of status, number of professional years, place of practice and speciality. Indeed, of the doctors who supported telemedicine, 47% were juniors and 53% seniors. This suggests that familiarity with digital technologies is not a determining factor in the adoption of telemedicine, as senior doctors are just as concerned as junior doctors.Similarly, our study showed that the interest shown in telepsychiatry did not vary according to speciality, since the majority of child psychiatrists surveyed expressed a favourable opinion. Certain characteristics linked to the interview in child psychiatry suggest that the interest in telepsychiatry in child psychiatry may be limited due to the use of mediation in play and motor skills, the need for specific teaching materials (toys, drawings, modelling clay) and the analysis of the child's movements in the room. In a study of psychiatrists in Normandy With regard to the practice of telepsychiatry, teleconsultation for children is the least envisaged in comparison with that for adolescents, adults and the elderly (18).

These data remain controversial, since other studies have shown the benefits of teleconsultation in children, and certain programmes dedicated to this population have revealed their feasibility, especially for neurodevelopmental disorders (19,20).The interest shown in telepsychiatry by the doctors surveyed supports the data collected worldwide, as shown by the experiences of several countries. Initially, telepsychiatry was only practised on an experimental and irregular basis in the United States between 1960 and 1970. Over the years, and thanks to rapid technological development, it has become a service tool for patients suffering from mental disorders in a number of countries around the world (21). Telepsychiatry is of particular interest in certain specific contexts, such as the shortage of psychiatrists, the shortage of care structures dedicated to mental disorders and the geographical remoteness of patients. This led the APA (the American Psychiatric Association) to recognise the value and place of telepsychiatry in the care of patients suffering from mental disorders, starting in 1998 (22).A review of the literature reveals numerous clinical demonstrations of telepsychiatry programmes. In other words, there is a growing number of controlled trials demonstrating the effectiveness of telepsychiatry in the specific treatment of several mental disorders and even in the management of crisis situations (23). For some groups of patients, the distance created by telepsychiatry may be seen as an advantage, as it may encourage their engagement with mental health care, particularly for patients with phobias or for the elderly subjects who may face obstacles such as reduced mobility, transport problems or social isolation (24,25). The effectiveness of psychiatry is far from being limited to traditional psychiatric treatment methods, and also extends to certain recent psychotherapeutic methods. One example is cognitive behavioural therapy (CBT) in the treatment of social phobia. In a recent meta-analysis including 42 articles, the results concluded that internet-based CBT was effective in the treatment of social phobia, with no significant difference compared with conventional CBT (26).

6. Legal and ethical issues surrounding telepsychiatry :

The first clinical vignette in this work raises the question of the practice of telemedicine in the context of a frequent psychiatric emergency, namely a high and eminent suicidal risk with a refusal on the part of the patient to be treated. In this situation, compulsory hospitalisation is indicated under article 11 of law 92/83 of 3 August 1992, reformed by law 40 of 3 May 2004, relating to mental health and conditions of hospitalisation for mental disorders (27).

The majority of doctors surveyed replied that it is necessary to contact the family in order to bring the patient to the psychiatric emergency department; although they know that the patient may refuse to go to the emergency department, may refuse to give us the contact details of family members, or the family may simply be unreachable. And it is in these critical, but at the same time fairly frequent, situations that the whole problem of medical responsibility lies when you choose to practise psychiatry at a distance.This situation raises questions about the psychiatrist's medical responsibility when managing a psychiatric emergency through teleconsultation. Should contact with the family be systematically maintained in high-risk situations and included in the electronic medical record? Should the Will telemedicine be able to trigger the procedure for compulsory hospitalisation? How can the psychiatrist contact the public prosecutor to report the need for compulsory hospitalisation? If the doctor refuses teleconsultation in this situation, or if the patient refuses to go to emergency and commits suicide, would the doctor be held medically liable for failing to assist a person in danger?

In what follows in this chapter, we will set out the ethical rules governing medical practice, with particular emphasis on the legal guarantees in telemedicine provided by the legislative decree. We will also examine certain legal issues relating to telemedicine, paying particular attention to its application in psychiatry.

6.1. Obligation to provide information and consent :

In the context of telemedicine, it is essential that each patient is informed of his or her state of health, the additional examinations requested, the treatments envisaged, their benefits and potential complications, the right to refuse or accept treatment, and also of the data relating to the consequences of using the technological device (accessibility, ease of use, risk). Doctors are responsible for providing clear, precise and appropriate information to each patient to enable them to make informed decisions about the care strategies that concern them (28).The fundamental principle of medical ethics, according to which the patient has a free choice of doctor, is set out in article 10 of the Tunisian Code of Medical Ethics (8). This principle may be restricted, particularly in the case of tele-expertise or tele-assistance. In these cases, the doctor must inform the patient of the need to seek the opinion of a colleague in the case of tele-expertise, or of another health professional (e.g. psychologist, second opinion from a psychiatrist) in the case of tele-assistance, and take his or her own decision.consent to exchange medical information through information technology as mentioned in article 23 of the presidential decree.Articles 19 and 21 of the decree-law reiterate these two obligations and state that information and consent must be recorded in the electronic medical record.

6.2. Confidentiality, safety and the obligation of medical secrecy:

In the present survey, around half the doctors replied that telepsychiatry increased the risk of disclosure of medical confidentiality.Protecting confidentiality is a legal obligation for doctors and must be respected in all situations, including when using modern communication technologies. According to article 254 of the Tunisian penal code and articles 8 and 9 of the code of medical ethics, doctors are obliged to guarantee the confidentiality of information to which they have access during the exercise of their profession (8,9).With telemedicine, the issue of confidentiality arises at two levels: during the telemedicine act itself and during the transfer and storage of data.

Article 22 of the decree-law specifies the nature of the data collected during telemedicine. In the same context, article 23 of the decree conditions the practice of telemedicine by mentioning the guarantees of security and confidentiality. The owner of the platform is prohibited from accessing this data, which can only be accessed by the requesting or requested doctor, or by the healthcare professionals taking part in the telemedicine procedure, after informing the patient and obtaining his or her consent.In addition, the technological system used constitutes a second level of concern in terms of confidentiality. Article 15 of the decree refers to technical and security requirements. Similarly, article 16 specifies that the data will be hosted in Tunisia by a national cloud service provider. The issue of archiving the electronic file was dealt with in the same article; the data will be transferred to and stored in a central database at the Ministry of Health's technical departments.The issue of confidentiality and medical secrecy is quite specific to psychiatry, especially in cases where the patient is incapable of consenting to treatment. In such cases, psychiatrists are sometimes obliged to inform the family in order to guarantee consultation and adherence to treatment. This can be a concern when practising telepsychiatry, which is not governed by legal or ethical rules.

6.3. Medico-legal liability and telemedicine :

Telemedicine creates new challenges and additional legal risks to those already present in traditional medical practice. The use of telemedicine raises complex legal issues that require particular attention, not only on the part of doctors, but also on the part of the various parties involved in the act of telemedicine (the treating doctor, the doctor required, the assistant doctor, the healthcare professional, the healthcare establishment and the IT support provider). In Tunisia, there is as yet no clearly defined legal or regulatory framework concerning the division of responsibilities between the various players involved in telemedicine, including third-party technology.In the event of a telecommunications system security failure, loss of data, hardware or software malfunction, or any other situation in which their product or service is considered to have caused damage, the supplier will be held liable. This is the liability of a technological third party.In this chapter, we are only going to look at the potential legal issues involved in acts relating to psychiatry, i.e. teleconsultation, tele-expertise and teleassistance.

6.3.1. Teleconsultation liability :

In teleconsultation, doctors are obliged to take great care in making their diagnosis, using all the means at their disposal. In terms of medical liability, the applicable regime is no different from that in force for a traditional consultation. The psychiatrist, like any other doctor using telemedicine during a consultation, may incur civil, criminal, administrative and disciplinary liability (29,30).

6.3.2. Responsibility in tele-expertise :

In telemedicine, liability may be incurred either by the requesting doctor, who will make the final decision, or by the requested doctor if he commits a fault, in particular by giving an opinion outside his field of expertise, omitting important elements or having technical problems.

Liability may also be shared if both doctors are at fault. In all cases, both professionals must act with probity and diligence, clarify situations that could affect their decisions and refrain from giving advice if necessary. Each practitioner assumes personal responsibility by applying the principle of obligation of means. The requested doctor must take into account the limits of the information and technologies used, seek additional expertise if necessary and clearly state the limits of his or her recommendation. He or she may also refuse to carry out the tele-expertise if, for example, he or she considers that the quality of the information is not sufficiently high.the medical information provided does not meet conventional image sharpness requirements. The requesting doctor is responsible for the information gathered and transmitted, the information given to the patient and the final decision regarding diagnosis or treatment (28-30).

6.3.3. Remote assistance liability :

As far as teleassistance is concerned, the liability applicable is the same as for teleconsultation or tele-expertise when medical acts are involved. In the diagnostic or therapeutic process, doctors share responsibility. When the teleassistance act is carried out, for example, between two psychiatrists and a psychologist. The second psychiatrist is responsible for the outcome of his assistance, while the psychologist is responsible for the diagnostic guidance he provides (29,30).

6.4. Liability and cross-border telemedicine :

The use of telemedicine can facilitate the practice of cross-border psychiatry, which raises additional legal issues. Issues of jurisdiction, regulation and compliance with the laws and standards of each country must be taken into account. It is worth mentioning that the principle of territoriality of laws means that the laws of the country where an offence is committed apply. This may pose difficulties in the event of a dispute involving a Tunisian doctor who may have made a mistake during a teleconsultation with a foreign patient who wishes to take legal action (28).

7. Ethical issues of telemedicine in psychiatry :

The second vignette presented in this work deals with the problem of announcing the diagnosis of a sexually transmitted infection contracted during a hypomanic episode in a patient being treated for bipolar disorder. The majority of doctors surveyed refused to inform patients by videoconference.The announcement of bad news must take account of certain ethical rules and good quality communication; in this particular case, the revelation of a severe diagnosis requires communication skills, an empathetic approach, detailed discussion and medical guidance. There is a risk that this framework will be disrupted during the videoconferencing announcement process, making the information difficult for the patient to understand or accept. The AETMIS recommendation advises against breaking bad news via telemedicine (10). In the present situation, it would be necessary to convert the teleconsultation into a face-to-face consultation, but this decision should in no way delay the announcement and management.The advent of a new technology should not lead to the creation of a new ethic, but it may require existing principles to be adapted to take account of the new situations it generates. Thus, the use of telemedicine in psychiatric practice may raise major ethical issues, and among the main fears raised, it will be legitimate to ask about the preservation of ethics and the future of the doctor-patient relationship.

7.1. Telepsychiatry and compliance with universal ethical principles :

According to our survey, 28% of doctors felt that telepsychiatry did not comply with universal ethical principles. The practice of telepsychiatry is still giving rise to reflection on its conformity with universal ethical principles, especially in the Tunisian context where the question of the feasibility of its application is quite new, and it is possible that its practice could be initiated in the near future.

- Charity :

Beneficence is a fundamental ethical principle in medicine. This principle implies that healthcare professionals have a moral obligation to do good and to act in the best interests of their patients. In telemedicine, this means that healthcare professionals must provide quality care at a distance, using appropriate technologies and complying with ethical and safety standards. It is essential that the quality of care provided by telepsychiatry is equivalent to that of conventional psychiatry. In its guide to good practice in telemedicine, the HAS urges doctors to be able to judge the relevance of a teleconsultation in the light of the patient's clinical situation, the availability of data and the patient's ability to communicate remotely and use IT tools (13).

In the absence of liaison psychiatry in many Tunisian hospitals, telepsychiatry may prove to be a viable solution for improving access to mental health care in the country. Similarly, in Tunisia, due to medical desertification, the shortage of mental health professionals and the relatively low density of psychiatrists in the country, telemedicine could play a crucial role in resolving this health crisis.

Similarly, in our socio-cultural context, mental disorders are still stigmatised and consulting a psychiatrist can be perceived negatively, telepsychiatry can help combat stigma by providing easier and more convenient access to mental healthcare for people who may be reluctant to visit a therapist in person (31). As a result, teleconsultation can offer a degree of anonymity and confidentiality.

- Non-maleficence :

As for the principle of non-maleficence, "Primum non nocere", this means that health professionals must assess the potential risks and benefits of their actions. of all medical interventions and take all necessary measures to prevent risks and negative side-effects for patients. In the context of telemedicine, certain precautions inherent in this new practice must be considered: security, confidentiality of medical records and respect for patient privacy. In the 2022 Ethics Manual, the WMA considered these requirements as duties towards the patient, and that the doctor should give priority to medical consultation and treatment through direct, personal contact where medically appropriate (12).

In Tunisia, the principle of non-maleficence may be restricted at the beginning of the use of this practice. This may be due to the fact that doctors are not trained and equipped in terms of knowledge and skills for the application of communication technologies. This lack of preparation may cause harm and damage in terms of confidentiality and the quality of care provided to patients, which could alter another ethical principle, namely professionalism. We believe that it will be desirable to ensure that the principle of professionalism is respected even before telemedicine is used.

- Autonomy :

Respect for autonomy is a fundamental ethical principle in medicine, stipulating that patients have the right to make decisions about their own health, based on their own judgement and value. The principle of respect for autonomy implies that patients must be fully informed about their state of health, the treatment options available, the risks and benefits of each option and their right to refuse or accept treatment (consent and information). In psychiatry, respecting patients' autonomy can be particularly complex because of mental disorders that may affect their ability to make informed decisions, or in psychiatric emergencies requiring coercive measures. Indeed, the issue of autonomy for patients suffering from mental disorders has given rise, and continues to give rise, to numerous ethical debates and reflections on this principle throughout the world. In telepsychiatry, the benefit/risk balance must be the subject of reflection for each patient, taking into account his or her particularities and pathology. In the light of these considerations, autonomy must be the rule for patients suffering from mental disorders, and the psychiatrist must involve the patient in his or her own care, while taking care to maintain an autonomous relationship outside risk situations that compromise this principle of autonomy and consent.

- Equity :

Equity is a fundamental ethical principle that requires all individuals to have equal access to healthcare. This means that every patient should have the opportunity to benefit from the same healthcare, without any discrimination based on origin, socio-economic status, age, gender or geographical location.

This principle may not be respected in telemedicine applied to psychiatry. Alternatively, telemedicine may act as a brake on the principle of equity in situations where it limits access to this care service for certain patients. For example, patients suffering from severe mental disorders, such as certain forms of schizophrenia or illnesses associated with profound neurocognitive disorders, may have difficulty using the Internet to communicate with their doctor (32).

On the other hand, in the Tunisian context, the principle of equity may be undermined by poor internet coverage in certain regions of the country. The fact that only 28% of the doctors surveyed have broadband access at their place of work highlights the logistical challenge involved in practising telepsychiatry. For telemental health, including telepsychiatry, to work effectively, it is necessary to have an internet connection. quality. According to AETMIS, the minimum threshold for adequate image and sound quality for psychiatric teleconsultations is 384 kbps (10)This speed is also recognised as minimal by the ATA, as the quality of the internet connection can affect the quality of the consultation and therefore the effectiveness of mental health care. The ATA has also issued recommendations for other factors such as bandwidth, camera position, lighting, monitor size and room environment, but these are not considered mandatory (11).At present, high and very high speed broadband is far from ubiquitous in Tunisia. According to the latest report from the International Telecommunications Union, the number of subscribers to fixed-line broadband access services will be 12.2 per 100 inhabitants in 2021, which raises the question of how to implement telemedicine from patients' homes (33).

7.2. Telepsychiatry and the doctor-patient relationship:

Around half the participants felt that telepsychiatry had a negative impact on the therapeutic relationship and risked dehumanising psychiatry.Telemedicine overturns a number of traditional principles governing the doctor-patient relationship, the basis on which therapeutic care is provided in the psychiatrist's day-to-day work. This relationship could be compromised by the fact that the use of ICTs is emerging as a third player in the doctor-patient relationship, making the interaction no longer binary but triangular. Furthermore, the use of telemedicine can lead to a certain dehumanisation of medicine because of the physical distance between doctor and patient, which can weaken the links between them. The fact that the doctor is virtual (e-medicine) can also lead to a situation where the patient is less inclined to listen to the doctor. Similarly, the doctor's empathy with a virtual patient (e-patient) is reduced. Therefore, to maintain a relationship of trust, it is necessary for the doctor and patient to have access to reliable mutual identification details for each telemedicine procedure (34).The fear of altering the quality of the psychiatric interview was identified by 35% of doctors. Indeed, the risk of losing non-verbal information (facial expression, gestures, body movements, eye contact and changes in tone of voice) during teleconsultation can alter therapeutic communication. For Van Wynsberghe and Gastamans, the psychiatrist's five senses must be called upon and the remote interview would only provide partial information to the patient, incompatible with quality care (35). With this in mind, some authors stress the need to maintain the doctor-patient relationship by combining face-to-face consultations if possible (34). Another socio-cultural issue that needs to be raised concerns the acceptance of telemedicine by Tunisian patients. For many of them, this method could be seen as a foreign form of care, which could lead to reluctance towards this new digital health culture and potentially affect the doctor-patient relationship.

8. Future prospects and recommendations :

In the light of our results and the data consulted, we can assume that Tunisian psychiatrists are committed to telemedicine and are aware of its benefits and what it can add to the care of patients with mental disorders in Tunisia. But the lack of knowledge about this practice and its recommendations, as well as the ethical and legal challenges it raises, may make it difficult to put into practice at this stage.

As a result, a number of recommendations can be drawn from these results:

- Set up specialised training programmes in telemedicine to improve knowledge of this new practice in Tunisia.

This training could cover theoretical knowledge, the different modalities and the technical and practical aspects of telemedicine, to help them make effective use of ICTs for remote care.

- Recognise the recommendations available in terms of telemedicine and advise practitioners of the need to comply with them.

- In order to achieve these first two objectives, theoretical courses and practical workshops can be integrated into the medical training curriculum at faculties of medicine, drawing on the experience of countries that have successfully integrated telemedicine into the continuum of care. These training programmes for students could involve a range of different people, including doctors, lawyers and IT specialists.

- Programme Masters Classes for doctors currently practising to raise their awareness of telemedicine and the issues it raises, and to promote new medical practices based on new technologies.

- Addressing the ethical issue of telemedicine in the various ethics committees in Tunisia in order to raise the main ethical issues at stake in the practice of remote medicine, but also to establish ethical guidelines guaranteeing a quality doctor-patient relationship.

- Define a legal framework for the division of responsibilities between the various players involved in telemedicine.

- Draw up a specific guide for psychiatrists on the best practice of telemedicine, taking into account the specific nature of this speciality.

- Defining care protocols for patients suffering from mental disorders, including telepsychiatry as a remote care option, adapting therapeutic programmes according to the nature of psychiatric disorders.

CONCLUSIONS

Telemedicine is becoming increasingly widespread in many countries, offering the possibility of providing medical care at a distance. This emerging mode of medical practice was particularly highlighted during the COVID-19 pandemic.In Tunisia, the legal framework for telemedicine was established by Law 2018-43 of 11 July 2018, which amended Law 91-21 of 13 March 1991 on the practice and organisation of the profession of doctor and dental practitioner. However, in order to specify the modalities of application of this practice, a presidential decree n° 318/2022 was published in the JORT on 8 April 2022.Because of certain particularities linked to its practice, psychiatry is one of the specialties most concerned by telemedicine. However, the intrusion of technology can disrupt certain traditional principles governing the therapeutic relationship and consequently have an impact on psychiatric care.The aim of this dissertation was to assess the knowledge, perceptions and support of Tunisian psychiatrists and child psychiatrists for telemedicine, while raising the ethical and medico-legal issues that could arise in our Tunisian context.A descriptive cross-sectional study was conducted 8 months after the publication of the presidential decree-law. The survey was conducted online using an electronic questionnaire designed on the Google Forms platform. The following were included: Tunisian psychiatrists and child psychiatrists practising in Tunisia in both the public and private sectors. The questionnaire was sent to 391 participants.During data collection, 70 participants answered the questionnaire, i.e. 17.9% of the doctors contacted by e-mail. Among these participants, two Tunisian doctors practising abroad were excluded. A total of 68 participants were included in this survey, divided into 50% senior doctors and 50% junior doctors.junior doctors (residents). Women predominated (78%; n=53). The median number of years in practice was 5±7 years. Of the participants, 82% (n=56) practised in psychiatry and 18% (n=12) in child psychiatry. The practice sector was public in 69% (n=47) and private in 31% (n=21) of cases. About half of the participants (53%; n=36) had a computer at work and only 28% (n=19) had broadband internet access (at least 384 kbps).The majority of them (62%; n=42) were not aware of the various telemedicine procedures and 57% (n=39) of doctors were not aware of the existence of Presidential Decree-Law No 318 / 2022 relating to the practice of telemedicine in Tunisia.The majority of doctors (81%; n=55) replied that telepsychiatry is more prone to legal problems than traditional psychiatry, and according to 49% telepsychiatry is more exposed to the risk of disclosure of medical confidentiality.Around half (56%; n=38) of doctors thought that telemedicine risked dehumanising the practice of psychiatry. Telepsychiatry alters the quality of the psychiatric interview according to 65% (n=44) of respondents, and has a negative impact on the quality of the doctor-patient relationship according to 43% (n=39). More than a third (28%; n=19) replied that telepsychiatry does not respect the ethical principles of medicine.The majority of doctors (84%) were in favour of telepsychiatry. No association was found between support for telepsychiatry and the status of the doctor (p=0.512), the number of years of professional experience (p=0.834) or his or her area of practice (p=1).Despite the interest in telemedicine among psychiatrists, our survey highlighted a lack of knowledge about this new mode of care.medical practice. The ethical and medico-legal issues addressed were the question of information, consent, the obligation of medical confidentiality and the right to quality care. We also raised the issue of medical liability in relation to the procedures most commonly used in telepsychiatry, namely teleconsultation, tele-expertise and teleassistance.The compliance of telepsychiatry with the ethical principles of medicine poses major challenges, particularly as regards respect for the principle of equity and beneficence. This is due to the nature of certain severe mental disorders, but also because of the logistical shortcomings and lack of ICT training among Tunisian doctors. Similarly, in the context of telepsychiatry, we have raised the question of the doctor-patient relationship, which with the use of ICT risks being reduced to a virtual relationship.Despite the current involvement of several Tunisian bodies and committees in promoting and developing e-health, such as CNT, INPDP, the Tunisian telemedicine and e-health society, digital health is coming up against several economic challenges (healthcare costs, health insurance systems), logistical and organisational challenges (digital infrastructure, internet access, IT equipment), as well as socio-cultural challenges (acceptance of digital culture, digital illiteracy), which can have an impact on the therapeutic relationship, trust, empathy and even the treatment of patients suffering from mental disorders.How can the psychiatrist and the Tunisian patient establish trust in IT tools? How can they see it as an effective ally in their therapeutic relationship?

REFERENCES

1. WHO Group Consultation on Health Telematics (1997: Geneva S. A health telematics policy in support of WHO's Health-for-all strategy for global health development: report of the WHO Group Consultation on Health Telematics, 11-16 December, Geneva, 1997 [Internet]. World Health Organization; 1998 [cited 2022 Dec 15]. Report No.: WHO/DGO/98.1. Available from: https://apps.who.int/iris/handle/10665/63857

2. Ohannessian R, Duong TA, Odone A. Global Telemedicine Implementation and Integration Within Health Systems to Fight the COVID-19 Pandemic: A Call to Action. JMIR Public Health Surveill. 2020;6(2):e18810.

3. Republic of Tunisia. Law No. 2018-43 of 11 July 2018, supplementing Law No. 91-21 of 13 March 1991, relating to the practice and organisation of the profession of doctor and dentist.Journal Officiel of 17 July 2018.

4. Republic of Tunisia. Law n° 91-21 of 13 March 1991, relating to the practice and organisation of the professions of doctor and dental practitioner. Official Journal of 15 March 1991.

5. Republic of Tunisia. Presidential decree n° 2022-318 of 8 April 2022, fixing the general conditions for the practice of telemedicine and the fields of its application. Official Journal of 17 April 2022.

6. Zgueb Y, Bourgou S, Neffeti A, Amamou B, Masmoudi J, Chebbi H, et al. Psychological crisis intervention response to the COVID 19 pandemic: A Tunisian centralised Protocol. Psychiatry Res. 2020;289:113042.

7. Mleyhi S, Ziadi J, Ben Hmida Y, Ghédira F, Ben Mrad M, Denguir R. Telemedicine and social networks in ECMO management in the era of COVID-19: the Tunisian experience. Ann CardiolAngeiol. 2021;70(2):125-8.

8. Republic of Tunisia. Tunisian Code of Medical Ethics. Decree no. 93-1155 of 17 May 1993, on the code of medical ethics of 1 June 1993.

9 Republic of Tunisia Code Pénal Tunisien. Available sur: https://www.ilo.org/dyn/natlex/docs/ELECTRONIC/61250/60936/F1198127290/TUN- 61250.pdf

10. Pineau G, Moqadem K, Saint-Hilaire C. Telehealth: clinical guidelines and technological standards in telepsychiatry. ETMIS. 2006;2(1):102.

11. Turvey C, Coleman M, Dennison O, Drude K, Goldenson M, Hirsch P, et al. ATA practice guidelines for video-based online mental health services. Telemed J E Health. 2013;19(9):722-30.

12 World Medical Association. WMA Policy Manual. Available at:

//www.wma.net/wp-content/uploads/2022/11/HB-F-Version-2022-2-2.pdf
13https://www.has-sante.fr/jcms/c_2971632/fr/teleconsultation-et-teleexpertise-guide-de-best practice

14. Elmatri A. Telemedicine in Tunisia: links with European, Arab and African countries. Tunisia: 4th International Conference: Sciences of Electronic, Technologies of Information and Telecommunications internet. March 2007. Available at: http://www.setit.rnu.tn/last_ edition/setit2007/T/2.pd
15. Brown FW. A survey of telepsychiatry in the USA. J Telemed Telecare. 1995;1(1):19-21.

16. Waseh S, Dicker AP. Telemedicine Training in Undergraduate Medical Education: Mixed- Methods Review. JMIR Med Educ. 2019;5(1):e12515.
17. Albarrak AI, Mohammed R, Almarshoud N, Almujalli L, Aljaeed R, Altuwaijiri S, et al. Assessment of physician's knowledge, perception and willingness of telemedicine in Riyadh region, Saudi Arabia. J Infect Public Health. 2021;14(1):97-102.
18. Thesis. Telemedicine in psychiatry: practices and representations among psychiatrists in Normandy
19. Doyen CM, Oreve MJ, Desailly E, Goupil V, Zarca K, L'Hermitte Y, et al. Telepsychiatry for Children and Adolescents: A Review of the PROMETTED Project. Telemed J E-Health Off J Am Telemed Assoc. 2018;24(1):3-10.
20. Kommu JVS, Sharma E, Ramtekkar U. Telepsychiatry for Mental Health Service Delivery to Children and Adolescents. Indian J Psychol Med. 2020;42(5 Suppl):46S-52S.
21. Shore J. The evolution and history of telepsychiatry and its impact on psychiatric care: Current implications for psychiatrists and psychiatric organizations. Int Rev Psychiatry Abingdon Engl. 2015;27(6):469-75.
American Psychiatric Association. Telepsychiatry Via Videoconferencing RESOURCE DOCUMENT. Available sur:
https://citeseerx.ist.psu.edu/document?repid=rep1&type=pdf&doi=8a483b3123f7110c46e4 3b242ab5d95658eb11b5
22. Astruc B, Henry C, Masson M. Interest of tele-psychiatry for patient management: issues and questions of a new practice. Ann Méd-PsycholRevPsychiatr. 2013;171(2):61-4.
23. Bouchard S, Paquin B, Payeur R, Allard M, Rivard V, Fournier T, et al. Delivering cognitive-behavior therapy for panic disorder with agoraphobia in videoconference. Telemed J E-Health Off J Am Telemed Assoc. 2004;10(1):13-25.

24. Desbordes M, Nebout S, Grès H, Guillin O, Haouzir S. Telemedicine in psychiatry of the elderly: challenges and prospects. NPG Neurol - Psychiatr - Gériatrie. 2015;15(89):270-3.
25. Romijn G, Batelaan N, Kok R, Koning J, van Balkom A, Titov N, et al. Internet-Delivered Cognitive Behavioral Therapy for Anxiety Disorders in Open Community Versus Clinical Service Recruitment: Meta-Analysis. J Med Internet Res. 2019;21(4):e11706.
26. Law no. 92-83 of 3 August 1992 on mental health and conditions of hospitalisation for mental disorders. Available at: https://legislation-securite.tn/en/law/44365#:~:text=Toute%20personne%20hospitalis%C3%A9e%20pour%20 des,l'%C3%A9tablissement%20d'hospitalisation.
27.Salem NH, Ouelha D, Gharbaoui M, Saadi S, Khelil MB. Medico-legal aspects of Telemedicine in Tunisia in the context of the Covid-19 pandemic. Tunis Med. 2020;98(6):423-33.
29- Williatte-Pellitteri L. Telemedicine and legal responsibilities. European Research in Telemedicine/La Recherche Européenne en Télémédecine 2013;2:17-22
30- Direction générale de l'offre de soins en France. Telemedicine and legal responsibilities engaged internet. 18 May 2012. Available at: https://solidarites-sante.gouv.fr/
31 Mejda C, Feten E, Anis Z, Afef L, Hedi A. History of the stigmatisation of the mentally ill in Tunisia. InfPsychiatr. 2007;83(8):689–94.
32. Välimäki M, Kuosmanen L, Hätönen H, Koivunen M, Pitkänen A, Athanasopoulou C, et al. Connectivity to computers and the Internet among patients with schizophrenia spectrum disorders: a cross-sectional study. Neuropsychiatr Dis Treat. 2017;13:1201-9.
33.World Bank Group. Subscriptions to fixed-line broadband access services (per100 inhabitants).at https://donnees.banquemondiale.org/indicateur/IT.NET.BBND.P2
34. Arné JL. Ethics, jurisprudence and telemedicine. Bull Acad Natl Med. 2014;198(1):119- 30.
35. vanWynsberghe A, Gastmans C. Telepsychiatry and the meaning of in-person contact: a preliminary ethical appraisal. Med Health Care Philos. 2009;12(4):469-76.

APPENDICES

Appendix 1: Questionnaire Socio-demographic and professional variables

1. Nationality: Tunisian, non-Tunisian

2. I currently work in Tunisia: yes, no

3. Gender: male, female

4. Age (in years)

5. Speciality: Psychiatry, Child psychiatry, Other

6. Number of years of professional experience (including residency) (in years)
7. Professional status: Resident, Specialist, Doctor, Assistant, Associate Professor, Professor
8. Practice sector: private, public

9. Location: rural or urban area

10. Average time taken to obtain a 1er consultation appointment: 2 weeks, 1 month, 3 months, more than 6 months
11. How to make an appointment : Paper diary, electronic diary, online electronic diary, on-site secretariat

12. Patients travelling more than 100 km (outward journey/return journey) to consult you Yes, No

13. Logistical impediment to consultation: yes, no

14. Reason for cancelling a consultation: Geographical distance, no means of transport, poses a somatic problem, work schedule constraint, patient travelling

Variables relating to the use of technological resources

1. Use of traditional technology (telephone, email, Facebook, social networks) in your professional practice: Yes, No
2. The main use of these means : Communicating with your patients, communicating with your patients' families, seeking advice from colleagues
3. Telephone intervention with patients in crisis: Yes, No
4. In your opinion, the impact of the intervention was: Positive, negative, neutral

5. Workplace equipment: Broadband Internet (at least 384 kbps), Computer, Camera, Microphone, Headset, Smartphone, Tablet, Other :

Variables relating to knowledge of telemedicine :

1. Knowledge of how telemedicine is applied (different telemedicine procedures): Yes , No
2. Knowledge of the definition of teleconsultation: yes, no
3. Knowledge of the definition of tele-expertise: yes, no
4. Knowledge of the definition of remote medical monitoring: yes, no
5. Knowledge of the definition of medical teleassistance: yes, no
6. Knowledge of the definition of medical regulation: yes, no
7. Electronic medical prescription: yes, no
8. Knowledge of the Presidential decree no.318/2022 on the use of telemedicine in Tunisia: yes, no
9. Knowledge of the procedure for practising telemedicine in Tunisia: yes, no
10. Knowledge of therecommendations practice of telemedicine/Telepsychiatry : Yes, No
11. Possibility of issuing medical prescriptions (Table B treatment; psychotropic drugs) via telemedicine: Yes, No
12. Possibility of practising telemedicine with a patient abroad: Yes, No

Variables relating to the interest in setting up future training in telepsychiatry :

1. The need for telemedicine training for psychiatrists: Yes, No
2. Priority of the content of this training: Methods of applying telemedicine (administrative, technical, recommendations for good practice), Ethical issues, Legal issues, etc.

Perception and usefulness of telepsychiatry in the Tunisian psychiatric care environment:

1. Usefulness of telepsychiatry in the Tunisian healthcare system: Yes, No
2. The telepsychiatry can facilitate access to care for patients being treated for a psychiatric disorder: Yes, No

3. Do you think that telepsychiatry concerns psychiatrists in free practice as well as university hospital psychiatrists: Yes, No
4. Do you think that telepsychiatry could be an alternative to the underdevelopment of liaison psychiatry? Yes, No
5. Usefulness of introducing telepsychiatry in Tunisian public hospitals : Yes , No
6. Can telepsychiatry make up for the shortage of psychiatrists in disadvantaged regions?
7. Usefulness of telepsychiatry for patients in prison: Yes, No
8. Telepsychiatry can be envisaged in : Adult psychiatry, child psychiatry, geriatric psychiatry
9. Telemedicine can be used : During psychiatric emergencies, as a first contact, during follow-up and monitoring (open question)
10. Telepsychiatry can be useful in the following areas: Addictology, psychotherapeutic techniques, suicide crisis management, cognitive remediation, other :

Ethical and medico-legal issues relating to telepsychiatry in Tunisia

1. Telepsychiatry alters the quality of the psychiatric interview: Yes, No
2. Telepsychiatry has a negative impact on the quality of the doctor-patient relationship: Yes, No
3. Telepsychiatry risks dehumanising the practice of psychiatry: yes, no
4. Do you think that telepsychiatry meets the ethical principles of medicine in the Tunisian context: Yes, No
5. In your opinion, what is the principle that telepsychiatry does not respect in our Tunisian context: Beneficence, Non-maleficence, Equity, Autonomy?
6. Telepsychiatry is more prone to forensic problems than traditional psychiatry: Yes, No
7. There is a greater risk of disclosure of medical confidentiality with telepsychiatry than with traditional psychiatry: Yes, No

Clinical vignettes :

- **Vignette 1:**

You are following a patient with bipolar disorder type 2, during the last hypomanic episode; he has had multiple sexual relationships, you ask for a serological test, the test comes back with an HIV+ serology. Would you agree to announce the diagnosis by teleconsultation: Yes, No

- **Vignette 2 :**

You are treating a patient who is having a suicidal crisis following a break-up, which you are unable to manage by teleconsultation. You suggest that she go to a psychiatric emergency department, but she refuses. What should you do?

Telepsychiatry membership :

Opinion on telepsychiatry: Favourable, Unfavourable

Appendix 2: Presidential Decree no. 2022-318 of 8 April 2022, laying down the general conditions for the practice of telemedicine and the areas of its application

Vu le décret n° 85-1216 du 5 octobre 1985, fixant les conditions d'intégration du personnel ouvrier dans le cadre des fonctionnaires,

Vu le décret n° 98-2509 du 18 décembre 1998, fixant le statut particulier au corps des ouvriers de l'Etat, des collectivités locales et des établissements publics à caractère administratif,

Vu le décret gouvernemental n° 2020-115 du 25 février 2020, fixant le statut particulier du corps administratif commun des administrations publiques,

Vu le décret Présidentiel n° 2021-137 du 11 octobre 2021, portant nomination de la Cheffe du Gouvernement,

Vu le décret Présidentiel n° 2021-138 du 11 octobre 2021, portant nomination des membres du Gouvernement,

Vu l'arrêté du Premier ministre du 4 mai 2010, fixant les modalités d'organisation de l'examen professionnel sur épreuves pour l'intégration des ouvriers appartenant à la catégorie dix dans le grade d'attaché d'administration du corps administratif commun des administrations publiques,

Arrête :

Article premier - Est ouvert au ministère de l'agriculture, des ressources hydrauliques et de la pêche maritime, le 30 mai 2022 et jours suivants, un examen professionnel sur épreuves pour l'intégration des ouvriers appartenant à la catégorie dix dans le grade d'administrateur adjoint du corps administratif commun des administrations publiques.

Art. 2 - Le nombre de postes à pourvoir est fixé à cinq (5) postes.

Art. 3 - La liste d'inscription des candidatures sera close le 29 avril 2022.

Art. 4 - Le présent arrêté sera publié au Journal officiel de la République tunisienne.

Tunis, le 5 avril 2022.

Le ministre de l'agriculture, des ressources hydrauliques et de la pêche maritime

Mahmoud Elyes Hamza

Vu

La Cheffe du Gouvernement

Najla Bouden Romdhane

MINISTERE DE LA SANTE

Décret Présidentiel n° 2022-318 du 8 avril 2022, fixant les conditions générales d'exercice de la télémédecine et les domaines de son application.

Le Président de la République,

Sur proposition du ministre de la santé,

Vu la Constitution et notamment ses articles 24 et 38,

Vu le décret Présidentiel n° 2021-117 du 22 septembre 2021, relatif aux mesures exceptionnelles,

Vu la loi organique n° 2004-63 du 27 juillet 2004, portant sur la protection des données à caractère personnel,

Vu la loi organique n° 2017-42 du 30 mai 2017, portant approbation de l'adhésion de la République tunisienne à la convention n° 108 du conseil de l'Europe pour la protection des personnes à l'égard du traitement automatisé des données à caractère personnel et de son protocole additionnel n° 181 concernant les autorités de contrôle et les flux transfrontières de données,

Vu la loi n° 69-54 du 26 juillet 1969, portant réglementation des substances vénéneuses, telle que modifiée et complétée par la loi n° 2009-30 du 9 juin 2009,

Vu la loi n° 73-55 du 3 août 1973, organisant les professions pharmaceutiques, ensemble les textes qui l'ont modifiée ou complétée et notamment la loi n° 2010-30 du 7 juin 2010,

Vu la loi n° 91-21 du 13 mars 1991, relative à l'exercice et à l'organisation de la profession de médecin et de médecin dentiste, telle que complétée par loi n° 2018-43 du 11 juillet 2018, et notamment son article 23 (bis),

Vu la loi n° 91-63 du 29 juillet 1991, relative à l'organisation sanitaire,

Vu la loi n° 2000-83 du 9 août 2000, relative aux échanges et au commerce électroniques, telle que modifiée par la loi organique n° 2004-63 du 27 juillet 2004,

Vu le code des télécommunications promulgué par la loi n° 2001-1 du 15 janvier 2001, ensemble les textes qui l'ont modifié ou complété et notamment la loi n° 2013-10 du 12 avril 2013,

Page 1058 — *Journal Officiel de la République Tunisienne* — **12 avril 2022** — N° 40

Vu la loi n° 2004-5 du 3 février 2004, relative à la sécurité informatique,

Vu la loi n° 2004-71 du 2 août 2004, portant institution d'un régime d'assurance maladie, telle que modifiée par la loi n° 2017-47 du 15 juin 2017,

Vu le décret-loi du chef du gouvernement n° 2020-31 du 10 juin 2020, relatif à l'échange électronique des données entre les structures et leurs usagers et entre les structures, ratifié par la loi n° 2021-14 du 7 avril 2021,

Vu le décret n° 73-259 du 31 mai 1973, portant code de déontologie dentaire, tel que complété par le décret n° 80-99 du 23 janvier 1980,

Vu le décret n° 74-1064 du 28 novembre 1974, relatif à la définition de la mission et des attributions du ministère de la santé,

Vu le décret n° 75-835 du 14 novembre 1975, portant code de déontologie pharmaceutique,

Vu le décret n° 79-735 du 22 août 1979, organisant le ministère de la défense nationale, ensemble les textes qui l'ont modifié ou complété et notamment le décret gouvernemental n° 2016-908 du 22 juillet 2016,

Vu le décret n° 80-1255 du 30 septembre 1980, portant statut particulier des médecins dentistes hospitalo-universitaires, ensemble les textes qui l'ont modifié ou complété et notamment le décret n° 2000-235 du 31 janvier 2000,

Vu le décret n° 81-1634 du 30 novembre 1981, portant règlement général intérieur des hôpitaux, instituts et centres spécialisés relevant du ministère de la santé,

Vu le décret n° 89-296 du 15 février 1989, fixant le statut du corps médical des hôpitaux, ensemble les textes qui l'ont modifié ou complété et notamment le décret n° 2001-316 du 23 janvier 2001,

Vu le décret n° 91-1844 du 2 décembre 1991, fixant l'organisation administrative et financière ainsi que les modalités de fonctionnement des établissements publics de santé, ensemble les textes qui l'ont modifié ou complété et notamment le décret gouvernemental n° 2016-569 du 13 mai 2016,

Vu le décret n° 93-1155 du 17 mai 1993, portant code de déontologie médicale, tel que complété par le décret gouvernemental n° 2018-34 du 10 janvier 2018,

Vu le décret n° 94-1744 du 29 août 1994, relatif aux modalités de contrôle technique à l'importation et à l'exportation et aux organismes habilités à l'exercer, ensemble les textes qui l'ont modifié ou complété et notamment le décret n° 2010-1684 du 5 juillet 2010,

Vu le décret n° 2001-318 du 23 janvier 2001, relatif à l'indemnité de garde et ses conditions d'attribution et fixant les taux de cette indemnité pour les personnels des corps médicaux et juxta médicaux hospitalo-universitaires et hospitalo-sanitaires et les médecins des hôpitaux exerçant dans les structures hospitalières et sanitaires publiques relevant du ministère de la santé publique ainsi que les résidents et les stagiaires internes en médecine, en pharmacie et en médecine dentaire, ensemble les textes qui l'ont modifié ou complété et notamment le décret gouvernemental n° 2019-773 du 30 août 2019,

Vu le décret n° 2005-3031 du 21 novembre 2005, fixant les modalités et les procédures de l'exercice du contrôle médical prévu par la loi n° 2004-71 du 2 août 2004, portant institution d'un régime d'assurance maladie,

Vu le décret n° 2005-3154 du 6 décembre 2005, portant détermination des modalités et procédures de conclusion et d'adhésion aux conventions régissant les rapports entre la caisse nationale d'assurance maladie et les prestataires de soins,

Vu le décret n° 2005-3295 du 19 décembre 2005, portant statut particulier des pharmaciens hospitalo-universitaires, tel que modifié et complété par le décret n° 2008-2754 du 4 août 2008,

Vu le décret n° 2005-3296 du 19 décembre 2005, portant statut particulier des pharmaciens hospitalo-sanitaires, tel que modifié et complété par le décret n° 2007- 2976 du 19 novembre 2007,

Vu le décret n° 2007-1367 du 11 juin 2007 portant détermination des modalités de prise en charge, procédures et taux des prestations de soins au titre du régime de base d'assurance maladie, tel que modifié par le décret n° 2008-756 du 24 mars 2008,

Vu le décret n° 2008-2638 du 21 juillet 2008, fixant les conditions de fourniture du service téléphonie sur protocole Internet, ensemble les textes qui l'ont modifié ou complété et notamment le décret n° 2014-2152 du 19 mai 2014,

Vu le décret n° 2008-3026 du 15 septembre 2008, fixant les conditions générales d'exploitation des réseaux publics des télécommunications et des réseaux d'accès, tel que modifié et complété par le décret n° 2014-53 du 10 janvier 2014,

Vu le décret n° 2008-3449 du 10 novembre 2008, fixant le statut particulier du corps médical hospitalo-sanitaire, tel que modifié par le décret gouvernemental n° 2019- 953 du 23 octobre 2019,

Vu le décret n° 2009-772 du 28 mars 2009, fixant le statut particulier du corps des médecins hospitalo-universitaires, tel que complété par le décret n° 2009-3353 du 9 novembre 2009,

Vu le décret n° 2009-2347 du 12 août 2009, relatif à la spécialisation en médecine dentaire et au statut juridique des résidents en médecine dentaire,

Vu le décret n° 2010-1668 du 5 juillet 2010, fixant les attributions et l'organisation des directions régionales de la santé,

Vu l'arrêté Républicain n° 2013-159 du 11 juin 2013, fixant le statut particulier du corps hospitalo-sanitaire militaire, ensemble les textes qui l'ont modifié ou complété et notamment le décret gouvernemental n° 2017-996 du 17 août 2017,

Vu le décret gouvernemental n° 2016-1066 du 15 août 2016, fixant les conditions et procédures d'émission des factures électroniques et de leur archivage,

Vu le décret gouvernemental n° 2016-1096 du 24 août 2016, portant organisation des structures sanitaires militaires,

Vu le décret gouvernemental n° 2018-230 du 8 mars 2018, fixant le statut particulier des internes en médecine et des résidents en médecine,

Vu le décret gouvernemental n° 2020-48 du 23 janvier 2020, relatif aux procédures d'homologation d'importation et de commercialisation des équipements terminaux de télécommunications et des équipements radioélectriques,

Vu le décret gouvernemental n° 2020-777 du 5 octobre 2020, fixant les conditions, les modalités et les procédures d'application des dispositions du décret-loi du chef du gouvernement n° 2020- 31 du 10 juin 2020, relatif à l'échange électronique de données entre les structures et leurs usagers et entre les structures,

Vu le décret Présidentiel n° 2021-137 du 11 octobre 2021, portant nomination de la Cheffe du Gouvernement,

Vu le décret Présidentiel n° 2021-138 du 11 octobre 2021, portant nomination des membres du Gouvernement,

Vu l'avis du ministre de l'intérieur,

Vu l'avis de l'Instance nationale de protection des données à caractère personnel,

Vu l'avis du Tribunal administratif.

Prend le décret Présidentiel dont la teneur suit :

Article premier - Les dispositions du présent décret Présidentiel fixent les conditions générales d'exercice de la télémédecine et les domaines de son application.

Chapitre premier

Dispositions générales

Art. 2 - Outre les dispositions de la loi n° 91-21 du 13 mars 1991, susvisée et celles du présent décret Présidentiel, l'exercice de la télémédecine est soumis aux dispositions des codes respectifs de déontologie médicale, du médecin dentiste et du pharmacien.

Art. 3 - Au sens du présent décret Présidentiel, on entend par :

- **La téléconsultation** : l'acte qui consiste, pour un médecin ou un médecin dentiste, à donner une consultation médicale à distance à un patient, éventuellement assisté d'un professionnel de santé qualifié.

- **La télé-expertise :** l'acte ayant pour objet de permettre à un médecin ou un médecin dentiste de solliciter à distance l'avis d'un ou plusieurs confrères, en raison de leurs formations ou de leurs compétences particulières, et ce sur la base d'informations médicales liées à la prise en charge d'un patient.

- **La télésurveillance médicale** : l'acte ayant pour objet de permettre à un médecin ou un médecin dentiste de surveiller et d'interpréter à distance les données nécessaires au suivi médical d'un patient et, le cas échéant, de prendre des décisions relatives à sa prise en charge. L'enregistrement et la transmission des données peuvent être automatisés ou réalisés par le patient lui-même ou par un professionnel de santé.

- **La téléassistance médicale :** l'acte ayant pour objectif de permettre à un médecin ou un médecin dentiste d'assister à distance un autre professionnel de santé lors de la réalisation d'un acte médical.

- **La régulation médicale :** la réponse médicale à distance apportée à un patient dans le cadre d'un tri médical pratiqué au niveau des services d'assistance médicale urgente afin de déterminer et d'enclencher la réponse la mieux adaptée à la nature de l'appel.

- **La prescription médicale électronique :** un document dématérialisé rédigé par un médecin ou un médecin dentiste dans le cadre de l'exercice de la télémédecine, déposé sur une plateforme sécurisée exprimant une décision médicale suite à l'examen du malade et qui comporte une prescription de médicaments, d'examens ou de soins. Elle doit comporter notamment l'identité du médecin ou du médecin dentiste, sa signature électronique, la date de l'examen et l'identité du patient.

- **La plateforme de télémédecine :** un bouquet de services numériques regroupés dans un espace commun dans le respect des règles d'urbanisation, d'interopérabilité, de sécurité et d'éthique permettant l'usage de services à valeur ajoutée dans le domaine de la télémédecine.

Art. 4 - La télémédecine est exercée par les médecins et médecins dentistes autorisés à exercer leur profession en Tunisie conformément à la législation et la réglementation en vigueur.

Chapitre II

Les domaines d'application de la télémédecine

Art. 5 - Constituent des actes de télémédecine, les actes de téléconsultation, de télé-expertise, de télésurveillance médicale, de téléassistance médicale et de régulation médicale.

Art. 6 - Sont fixées par arrêté du ministre chargé de la santé les conditions spécifiques de la réalisation des actes de télémédecine pour chaque spécialité médicale ou chirurgicale.

Les conditions spécifiques de la réalisation des actes de télémédecine pour les spécialités techniques médicales militaires sont fixées par arrêté du ministre chargé de la santé, après avis du ministre chargé de la défense nationale.

Art. 7 - La réalisation des actes de télémédecine dans les deux secteurs public et privé s'effectue dans le cadre d'une plateforme ou d'un projet de coopération médicale entre les structures sanitaires publiques, entre une structure sanitaire publique et une autre structure publique ou entre une structure sanitaire publique et un établissement sanitaire privé.

Les modalités de coopération médicale entre les structures et établissements visés à l'alinéa premier du présent article pour la réalisation des actes de télémédecine sont fixées dans le cadre d'une convention conclue à cet effet entre les structures concernées.

Chapitre III

Les conditions générales d'exercice de la télémédecine

Section I - **L'autorisation**

Art. 8 - La réalisation des actes de télémédecine est soumise, outre l'autorisation de l'Instance nationale de protection des données à caractère personnel, à une autorisation préalable du ministère de la santé octroyée conformément aux procédures définies par le présent décret Présidentiel, après avis d'un comité d'évaluation dont les attributions, la composition et les modalités de fonctionnement sont fixées par arrêté du ministre de la santé.

Sous réserve des dispositions de l'alinéa premier du présent article, la réalisation des actes de télémédecine dans le milieu militaire peut être soumise à des procédures spécifiques fixées par arrêté du ministre de la défense nationale.

Art. 9 - Toute personne désirant mettre en place une plateforme de télémédecine ou réaliser des actes de télémédecine dans le cadre d'un projet de coopération médicale, doit déposer, auprès du ministère de la santé, une demande contre décharge indiquant la date de dépôt de la demande ainsi que la liste des documents déposés.

Le comité visé à l'article 8 du présent décret Présidentiel, doit, dés la réception de la demande d'autorisation, vérifier qu'il contient tous les documents définis par arrêté du ministre de la santé. Si la demande est incomplète, le comité doit, dans un délai maximal de vingt (20) jours ouvrables, à compter de la date du dépôt de la demande, convoquer le demandeur de l'autorisation, par tout moyen laissant une trace écrite, pour compléter son dossier.

Art. 10 - Le ministère chargé de la santé doit répondre aux demandes d'autorisation de la mise en place de la plateforme de télémédecine ou de l'exercice des actes de télémédecine dans le cadre d'un projet de coopération médicale dans un délai maximum de quatre vingt dix (90) jours à compter de la date de dépôt d'un dossier complet.

En cas de refus, la décision de refus doit être écrite et motivée.

Art. 11 - L'utilisation de la plateforme de télémédecine se fait par une convention conclue à cet effet entre le propriétaire de la plateforme et le médecin ou le médecin dentiste concerné.

Pour les médecins et les médecins dentistes de libre pratique, la convention doit être visée par l'ordre professionnel concerné qui se charge d'en informer le ministère de la santé dans un délai ne dépassant pas trente (30) jours de la date de conclusion de ladite convention.

Pour les médecins et les médecins dentistes exerçant dans le secteur public, la convention doit être visée par le ministère de tutelle sectorielle concerné.

L'exercice de télémédecine dans le cadre d'un projet de coopération médicale se fait soit par l'utilisation des moyens propres de l'établissement ou par un contrat conclu, à cet effet, entre le représentant légal de l'établissement et le propriétaire de la plateforme.

Le modèle de la convention et du contrat visés aux alinéas 1 et 2 du présent article est fixé par arrêté du ministre de la santé.

Art. 12 - La demande d'autorisation de la mise en place de la plateforme de télémédecine doit contenir une présentation détaillée des frais d'utilisation envisagés pour les différentes catégories d'utilisateurs.

Les frais résultant de l'utilisation de la plateforme de télémédecine sont fixés de manière à garantir un accès équitable aux services de télémédecine par les professionnels de santé et ce indépendamment du nombre d'actes réalisés.

Aucun frais n'est exigé lors de l'utilisation des pharmaciens de la plateforme de télémédecine pour assurer la dispensation des médicaments sur prescription médicale électronique.

Art. 13 - L'exercice de la télémédecine, destiné aux patients résidents à l'étranger, par les médecins et les médecins dentistes relevant du secteur public ou du secteur privé, doit être déclaré préalablement aux services compétents du ministère de la santé et aux ordres professionnels concernés.

Section II - **Les conditions techniques**

Art. 14 - La plateforme de télémédecine et le projet de coopération médicale, doivent répondre aux exigences techniques de qualité et de sécurité requises.

La plateforme de télémédecine, ne doit, en aucun cas, constituer un support publicitaire pour les produits de santé ou un moyen orientant les patients vers tout prestataire de service de santé.

Art. 15 - Les exigences techniques et les exigences de sécurité des moyens utilisés dans la réalisation des actes de télémédecine et de conservation des données collectées sont fixées par arrêté conjoint des ministres chargés de la santé et des technologies de la communication.

L'importation des outils individuels d'enregistrement et de transmission des données, utilisés par les patients est soumise à une autorisation de mise à la consommation conformément à la législation et la règlementation en vigueur.

Art. 16 - Les données traitées dans le cadre des actes de télémédecine, doivent être hébergées et stockées en Tunisie chez un prestataire de services Cloud et hébergement national conformément à la législation et la règlementation en vigueur en matière de sécurité informatique et de protection des données à caractère personnel.

L'accès aux données visées à l'alinéa premier du présent article se fait conformément à la législation en vigueur.

Les données relatives aux actes de télémédecine doivent être instantanément transférées et conservées dans le dossier médical électronique du patient stocké au niveau d'une base de données centrale auprès des services techniques relevant du ministère de la santé. Les caractéristiques techniques du dossier médical électronique sont fixées par arrêté conjoint des ministres chargés de la santé et des technologies de la communication.

Les données traitées dans le cadre des actes de télémédecine effectués aux structures et établissements relevant du ministère de la défense nationale sont hébergées, conservées et transférées au niveau d'une base de données spécifique.

Art. 17 - Les versions numériques des comptes-rendus et des prescriptions médicales issues d'un acte de télémédecine doivent être renforcées par une signature électronique conformément à la législation et à la règlementation en vigueur.

Art. 18 - Les pharmaciens titulaires d'officines de détail peuvent, dans le cadre des actes de télémédecine, dispenser les médicaments, au public, hormis les médicaments du tableau B et les psychotropes soumis au contrôle du ministère de la santé, et ce sur prescription médicale électronique moyennant l'utilisation d'un système d'information sécurisé garantissant la protection, la sécurité et la fiabilité des documents et des données personnelles conformément à la législation en vigueur.

Les conditions et les modalités de dispensation de la prescription médicale électronique sont fixées par arrêté du ministre de la santé.

Section III - **Les garanties de l'exercice de la télémédecine**

Art. 19 - La réalisation de tout acte de télémédecine doit être effectuée dans un cadre garantissant :

- l'identification du patient moyennant l'utilisation d'un système d'information fiable et sécurisé,

- l'authentification des professionnels de santé participant à l'acte de télémédecine,

- l'information du patient de l'identité des professionnels de santé participant à l'acte de télémédecine,

- la qualité des soins et des actes médicaux fournis,

- l'accès nécessaire du professionnel de santé, selon la nature de son intervention, aux données médicales du patient, nécessaires pour la réalisation de l'acte de télémédecine,

- la préservation du secret médical relatif à la réalisation de l'acte de télémédecine,

- la possibilité, pour le malade, de s'abstenir à continuer le traitement à distance et de choisir un autre mode de soins,

- la conformité de la plateforme et de tous les outils informatiques utilisés à la législation en vigueur relative notamment à la sécurité informatique et à la protection de données à caractère personnel,

- la traçabilité de toutes les informations relatives à l'acte de télémédecine, et la conservation des données à caractère personnel pendant dix (10) ans, au moins. Ces données doivent être accessibles, après consentement du patient ou de son tuteur légal, au cas où le patient fait appel à un autre médecin pour faire un acte de télémédecine,

- l'interopérabilité, le transfert, l'échange et la réversibilité des données collectées, et ce, dans le cadre d'un standard qui permet leur exploitation par d'autres structures professionnelles responsables et/ou d'autres plateformes dûment autorisées,

- l'accès aux informations relatives à l'acte de télémédecine par les organes de contrôle et d'inspection dûment qualifiés.

Art. 20 - Les conditions et les modalités d'échange électronique des données entre les propriétaires de la plateforme de télémédecine et la caisse nationale d'assurance maladie, sont fixées dans le cadre des conventions conclues à cet effet entre les parties. Les dites conventions entrent en vigueur après leur approbation par arrêté du ministre chargé des affaires sociales.

Art. 21 - Avant la réalisation de tout acte de télémédecine, le consentement libre et éclairé du patient ou, le cas échéant, de son tuteur légal doit être recueilli et ce après son information de la nécessité, de l'intérêt, des conséquences et de la portée dudit acte ainsi que des moyens mis en œuvre pour sa réalisation.

L'information et le consentement libre et éclairé du patient ou de son tuteur légal doivent être matérialisés par tout moyen laissant une trace sur un support électronique et, au besoin, papier.

Art. 22 - Les données à caractère personnel du patient relatives à la santé recueillies lors de la réalisation d'un acte de télémédecine doivent être inscrites sous forme d'un rapport détaillé contenant, notamment, les informations suivantes :

- les données médicales relatives au patient, les actes médicaux réalisés et les prescriptions médicales rédigées à cet effet,

- l'identification des professionnels de santé impliqués dans la réalisation de l'acte de télémédecine,

- La date et l'heure de la réalisation de l'acte de télémédecine.

- Les incidents techniques éventuels survenus.

Les données susvisées ne sont accessibles à d'autres professionnels de santé qu'après autorisation explicite du patient.

Sous réserve de la législation en vigueur, est interdite au propriétaire de la plateforme de télémédecine, l'utilisation ou la gestion des données personnelles des malades relatives à la santé, recueillies lors de la réalisation des actes de télémédecine.

Art. 23 - Sous réserve de la législation et de la règlementation en vigueur relatives à la protection des données à caractère personnel, les professionnels de santé participant à la réalisation d'un acte de télémédecine doivent avoir le consentement de la personne concernée dudit acte, dûment informée, pour échanger les informations qui le concernent, notamment par le biais des technologies de l'information et de la communication.

Section IV - **Les modalités de paiement et de rémunération des actes de télémédecine**

Art. 24 - La tarification et les modalités de paiement des actes de télémédecine concernés par les dispositions du présent décret Présidentiel, sont fixés par arrêté conjoint des ministres chargés de la santé, des affaires sociales et des finances, après avis des ordres professionnels concernés.

La rémunération des actes de télémédecine réalisés dans le secteur public se fait conformément aux dispositions du décret n° 2001-318 du 23 janvier 2001, susvisé.

Art. 25 - Les tarifications des actes de télémédecine à destination de patients résidents à l'étranger, effectués par les professionnels de santé relevant du secteur public sont fixées dans le cadre des conventions établies à cet effet par les structures et les établissements sanitaires concernés.

Les tarifications des actes de télémédecine à destination de patients résidents à l'étranger, effectués par les professionnels de santé de libre pratique sont fixée dans le cadre des conventions établies à cet effet et qui doivent être visées par l'ordre professionnel concerné.

Chapitre IV

Dispositions finales et transitoires

Art. 26 - L'autorisation pour l'utilisation de la plateforme de télémédecine ou pour l'exécution du projet de coopération médicale est retirée par arrêté du ministre de la santé, en cas d'inobservation, dûment constatée, des exigences requises par les services compétents du ministère de la santé ou des autres ministères de tutelle sectorielle. L'autorisation est retirée temporairement ou définitivement.

Art. 27 - A titre exceptionnel et dans le cadre de la mobilisation des ressources humaines nécessaires pour faire face à la propagation du virus SARS-Cov2, et pour une période ne dépassant pas un an à compter de la date de publication du présent décret Présidentiel au Journal officiel de la République tunisienne, les téléconsultations au profit des personnes infectées par le Virus suivies à domicile ou après leur hospitalisation, sont assurées à titre gratuit.

La période visée à l'alinéa premier du présent article peut être prolongée, par arrêté du ministre de la santé, pour une durée allant de six (6) mois à un an et ce en fonction de l'évolution de la situation épidémique dans le pays.

Les médecins et les médecins dentistes tunisiens exerçant à l'étranger peuvent, pendant la même période, dans le cadre d'échanges d'expertise et pour faire face à la propagation du virus SARS-Cov2, être autorisés par le ministre de la santé, après avis des organismes professionnels concernés, à effectuer les actes de téléconsultation et ce à titre gratuit, à travers une plateforme dûment autorisée à cet effet en Tunisie.

Art. 28 - Les propriétaires des plateformes de télémédecine et les responsables des projets de coopération médicale en activité à la date de parution du présent décret Présidentiel, sont tenus de se conformer à ses dispositions dans un délai ne dépassant pas un an à compter de la date de son entrée en vigueur.

Art. 29 - Le présent décret Présidentiel sera publié au Journal officiel de la République tunisienne.

Tunis, le 8 avril 2022.

Pour Contreseing
La Cheffe du Gouvernement
Najla Bouden Romdhane

Le ministre de la santé
Ali Mrabet

Le ministre de la défense nationale
Imed Memiche

La ministre des finances
Sihem Boughdiri Nemsia

Le ministre des affaires sociales
Malek Zahi

Le ministre des technologies de la communication
Nizar Ben Neji

Le Président de la République
Kaïs Saïed

Appendix 2: Approval of the Ethics Committee

REPUBLIQUE TUNISIENNE
MINISTERE DE LA SANTE
HOPITAL RAZI-2010 LA MANNOUBA
LE COMITE D'ETHIQU

Présidente Pr. R. LABBANE

DECISION RP B 01/2023

Le comité éthique de l'hopital Razi a été saisi par le résident Samaâli Samir pour une demande d'avis concernant le travail de Mémoire :

La télémédecine en psychiatrie : enjeux et questions d'une nouvelle pratique en Tunisie.

Le comité a examiné les documents suivants:

° Méthodologie détaillée de l'étude

Le comité a adopté la décision suivante : Favorable

Date de l'avis : 4/4/23

Signature de la Présidente du comité d'Ethique

SUMMARY

Introduction :

In Tunisia, the legal framework governing the practice of telemedicine was recently defined by Presidential Decree-Law No. 318/2022 of 8 April, published in the Journal Officiel de la République Tunisienne. Psychiatry is one of the specialties most concerned by this new medical practice.The objectives of this study were to assess the knowledge, perception and acceptance of telemedicine among Tunisian psychiatrists and child psychiatrists, and to raise the ethical and medicolegal issues that may arise from the practice of telemedicine in psychiatry in the Tunisian context.

Methods :

A descriptive cross-sectional study was conducted 8 months after the publication of the presidential decree. The survey was conducted online using an electronic questionnaire designed on the Google Forms platform. The questionnaire was sent to 391 Tunisian psychiatrists and child psychiatrists practising in Tunisia in both the public and private sectors.

Results :

A total of 68 participants were included in this survey. The median number of years of professional experience was 5±7 years. Of the participants, 82% (n=56) practised in psychiatry and 18% (n=12) in child psychiatry. The practice sector was public in 69% (n=47) and private in 31% (n=21) of cases. The majority (62%; n=42) were not aware of the various telemedicine procedures, and 57% (n=39) of doctors were not aware of the existence of the decree-law. The majority of doctors (81%; n=55) replied that telepsychiatry is more prone to legal problems than traditional psychiatry, and according to 49% (n=33), telepsychiatry is more exposed to the risk of disclosure of medical confidentiality. Around half (56%; n=38) of doctors thought that telemedicine risked dehumanising the practice of psychiatry. More than a third (28%; n=19) replied that telepsychiatry does not respect the ethical principles of medicine. The majority of doctors (84%,n=57) were in favour of telepsychiatry.

Conclusion:

The results of the study testify to the interest of Tunisian psychiatrists in telemedicine, while highlighting a lack of knowledge about this emerging medical practice. The ethical and legal challenges raised by telemedicine in psychiatry may make it difficult to implement for the time being.

Key word : Telemedicine, Psychiatry, Legal aspects, Ethical issues, Attitude, Tunisia

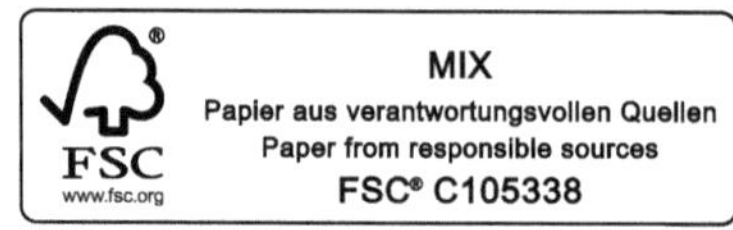

Printed by Books on Demand GmbH, Norderstedt / Germany